40ish WEEKS
a pregnancy journal

created & illustrated by
Kate Pocrass

CHRONICLE BOOKS
SAN FRANCISCO

ISBN 978-1-4521-3915-9

Manufactured in China

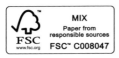

Designed by Kate Pocrass
See the full range of Kate Pocrass gift products at
www.chroniclebooks.com

10 9 8 7 6

Chronicle Books LLC
680 Second Street
San Francisco, CA 94107
www.chroniclebooks.com

CONGRATS
so the adventure begins

A whole lot can happen in just 40ish weeks. All of a sudden there are mood swings, cravings, moments of sheer amazement, and overwhelming emotions. Not to mention the breakouts, nights of restlessness, expanding belly, hidden toes, and ever-growing list of advice you get from friends, family, doctors — even strangers.

With so much going on, it can be hard to keep track of everything you're experiencing. Let **40ish Weeks** be your guide through it all. The journal is organized by trimester, but since every pregnancy moves at its own pace, you can jump ahead or return to any page when fitting. You'll find places to document all the little details so that nothing goes unrecorded. For each beautiful moment of pregnancy, there are a handful of unglorified moments that will be just as fun to look back on. The everyday minutiae of pregnancy are often what give you the truest glimpse of this momentous time in your life.

Remember to sit back, take note, and reflect on all that happens in these unbelievable weeks. In the end you will create a funny, lighthearted snapshot of your pregnancy to look back on for years to come.

—Kate Pocrass

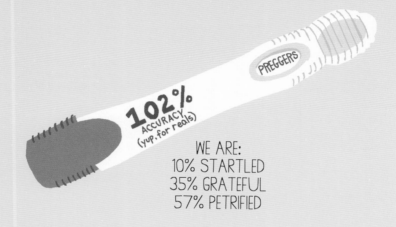

102%
ACCURACY
(yup, for reals)

WE ARE:
10% STARTLED
35% GRATEFUL
57% PETRIFIED

PREGGERS

1st
trimester

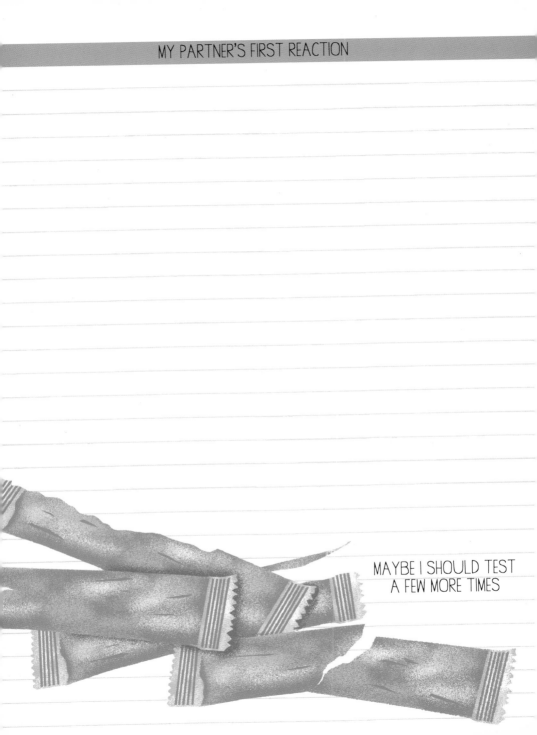

MAYBE I SHOULD TEST
A FEW MORE TIMES

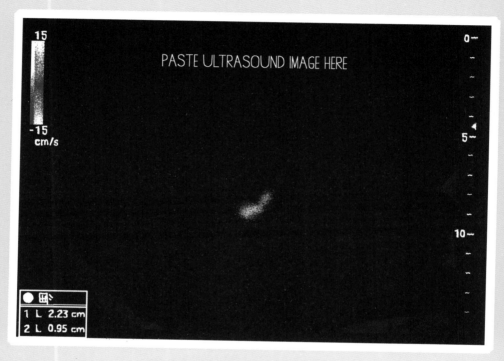

AND SOMEHOW YOU INSTANTLY
FALL IN LOVE WITH A BLOB

- [ ]
- [ ]
- [ ]
- [ ]
- [ ]
- [ ]
- [ ]
- [ ]
- [ ]
- [ ]
- [ ]
- [ ]
- [ ]
- [ ]
- [ ]

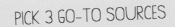

SIFTING THROUGH THE INFORMATION OVERLOAD

PICK 3 GO-TO SOURCES

BAN ONLINE FORUMS

RESIST URGE TO LOOK UP
EVERY SYMPTOM

DOCTOR KNOWS MORE THAN
RANDOM INTERNET SEARCH

GET 1 REALLY GOOD BOOK

GET 1 REALLY GOOD APP

PREGNANCY-RELATED IMAGE
SEARCHES ARE OFTEN WEIRD

TRUSTED WEBSITES & APPS

- [ ] ....
- [ ] ....
- [ ] ....
- [ ] ....
- [ ] ....
- [ ] ....
- [ ] ....
- [ ] ....
- [ ] ....
- [ ] ....
- [ ] ....
- [ ] ....
- [ ] ....
- [ ] ....
- [ ] ....
- [ ] ....
- [ ] ....
- [ ] ....
- [ ] ....
- [ ] ....
- [ ] ....
- [ ] ....
- [ ] ....
- [ ] ....
- [ ] ....

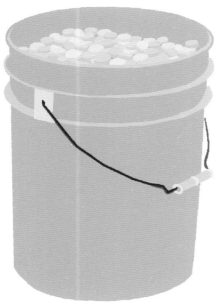

IT'S A SHAME THEY DON'T
SELL ANTACID IN BULK

EARLY PREGNANCY SYMPTOMS

- [ ] ....
- [ ] ....
- [ ] ....
- [ ] ....
- [ ] ....
- [ ] ....
- [ ] ....
- [ ] ....
- [ ] ....
- [ ] ....
- [ ] ....
- [ ] ....
- [ ] ....
- [ ] ....
- [ ] ....
- [ ] ....
- [ ] ....
- [ ] ....
- [ ] ....
- [ ] ....
- [ ] ....
- [ ] ....
- [ ] ....
- [ ] ....
- [ ] ....
- [ ] ....

FOOD AVERSIONS

- [ ]
- [ ]
- [ ]
- [ ]
- [ ]
- [ ]
- [ ]
- [ ]
- [ ]
- [ ]
- [ ]

THINGS THAT KEEP THE BELLY CALM

- [ ]
- [ ]
- [ ]
- [ ]
- [ ]
- [ ]
- [ ]
- [ ]
- [ ]
- [ ]
- [ ]

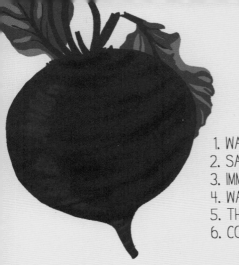

1. WALKED TO STORE
2. SAW BEETS IN SOMEONE'S CART
3. IMMEDIATELY NEEDED TO EAT BEETS
4. WALKED HOME
5. THOUGHT ABOUT THE SMELL OF COOKED BEETS
6. COULD NOT BEAR TO COOK BEETS

- ....
- ....
- ....
- ....
- ....
- ....
- ....
- ....
- ....
- ....
- ....
- ....
- ....
- ....
- ....
- ....
- ....
- ....
- ....
- ....
- ....
- ....
- ....
- ....
- ....
- ....

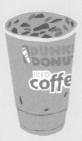

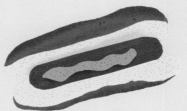

NOT EVEN AT THE
BALLPARK?

NO DIPPY EGGS?

OW AM I SUPPOSED TO
GET THROUGH THIS?

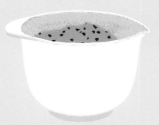

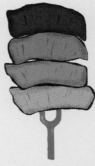

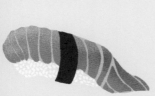

COOKED SUSHI IS NO
SUBSTITUTE

HOW CAN COOKIE
DOUGH BE WRONG?

WELL DONE?
WHY EVEN BOTHER?

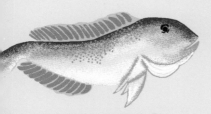

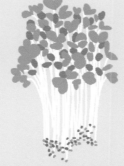

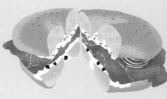

KAY, I DIDN'T LIKE MERCURY
MUCH ANYWAY

I THOUGHT THEY WERE
SO HEALTHY

SUNDAY MORNING
TRADITION ON HIATUS

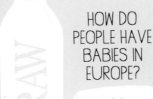

HOW DO
PEOPLE HAVE
BABIES IN
EUROPE?

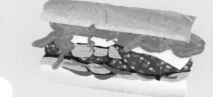

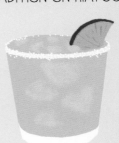

WHAT WILL I SUB
FOR MY SUB?

VIRGIN MARGARITA,
WHAT IS THE POINT?

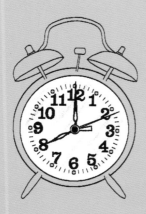

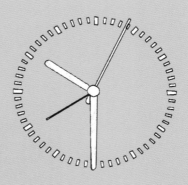

WAKE UP AT 8 a.m. – EXHAUSTED BY 10:30 a.m.

☐ NEED CONSTANT CATNAPS
☐ HARD TO HOLD HEAD UPRIGHT
☐ TOO TIRED TO STAY ALIVE

I THOUGHT I HAD MOVED BEYOND PIMPLES

- [ ] ....
- [ ] ....
- [ ] ....
- [ ] ....
- [ ] ....
- [ ] ....
- [ ] ....
- [ ] ....
- [ ] ....
- [ ] ....
- [ ] ....
- [ ] ....
- [ ] ....
- [ ] ....
- [ ] ....
- [ ] ....
- [ ] ....
- [ ] ....
- [ ] ....
- [ ] ....
- [ ] ....
- [ ] ....
- [ ] ....
- [ ] ....
- [ ] ....

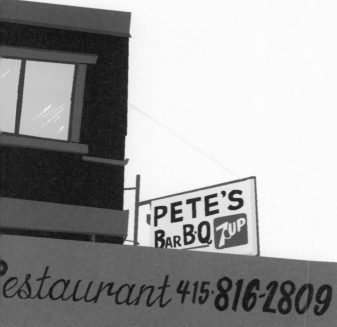

DRIVE 2 BLOCKS OUT OF MY WAY
TO AVOID THE PREVIOUSLY WELCOME
SMELL OF ROASTING CHICKENS

WAYS TO HIDE THAT I AM PREGNANT

- [ ]
- [ ]
- [ ]
- [ ]
- [ ]
- [ ]
- [ ]
- [ ]
- [ ]
- [ ]
- [ ]
- [ ]
- [ ]
- [ ]
- [ ]
- [ ]
- [ ]
- [ ]
- [ ]
- [ ]
- [ ]
- [ ]
- [ ]
- [ ]
- [ ]
- [ ]
- [ ]

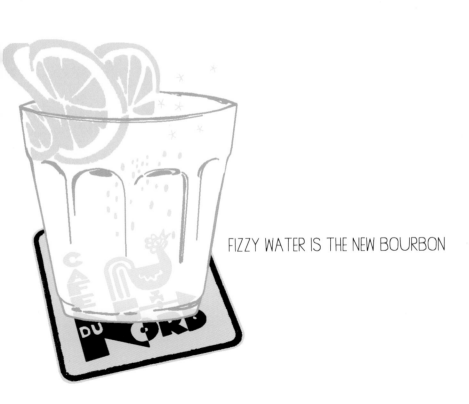

FIZZY WATER IS THE NEW BOURBON

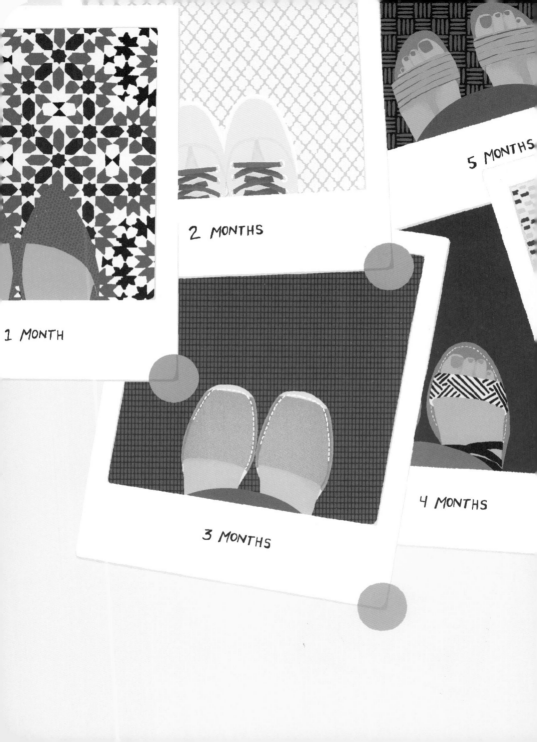

1 MONTH

2 MONTHS

3 MONTHS

4 MONTHS

5 MONTHS

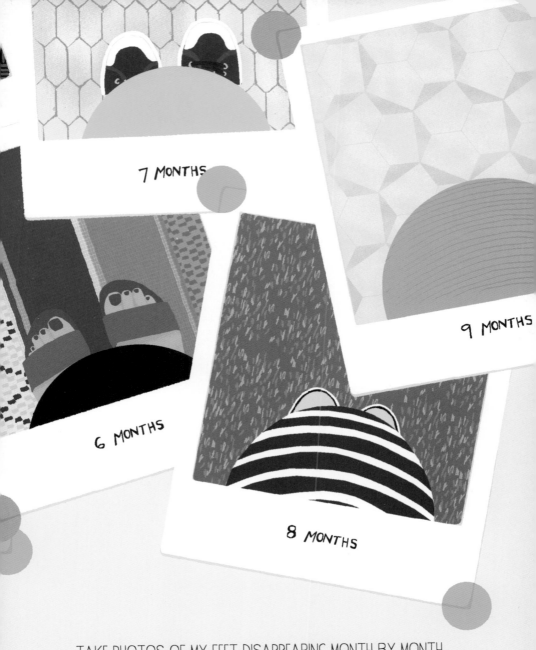

7 MONTHS

9 MONTHS

6 MONTHS

8 MONTHS

TAKE PHOTOS OF MY FEET DISAPPEARING MONTH BY MONTH

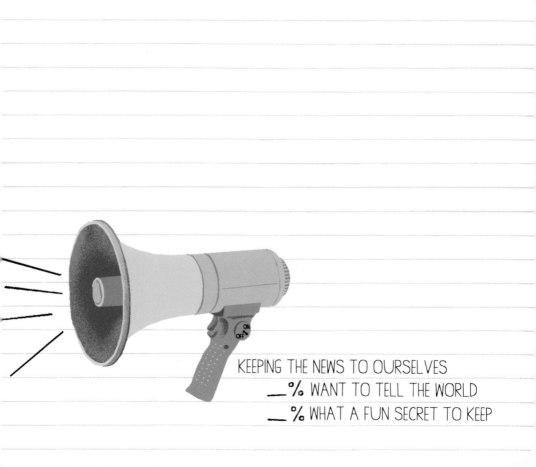

KEEPING THE NEWS TO OURSELVES
___% WANT TO TELL THE WORLD
___% WHAT A FUN SECRET TO KEEP

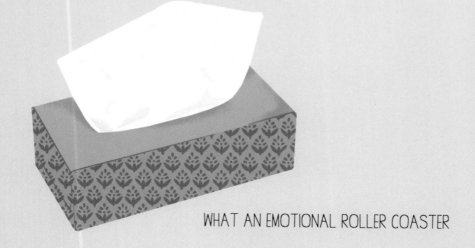

WHAT AN EMOTIONAL ROLLER COASTER

☐ HAPPIEST WOMAN IN THE WORLD
☐ GOING TO CRY ANY MINUTE NOW
☐ SEVERE CASE OF ROAD RAGE

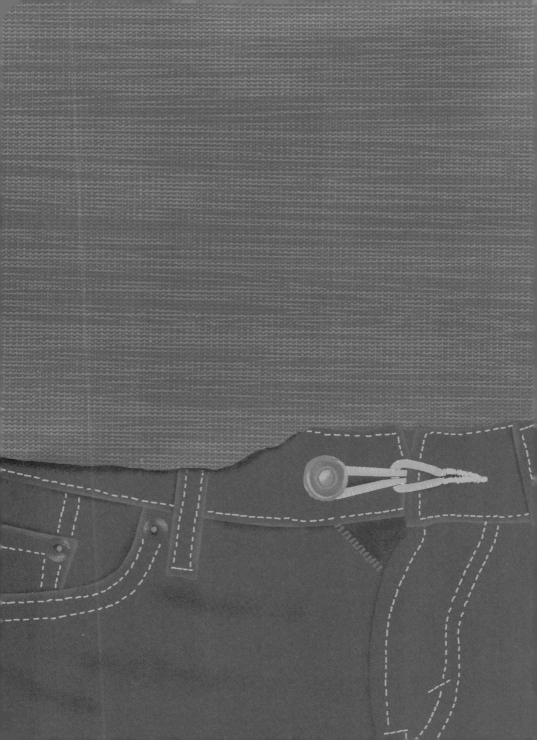

IT'S TIME TO
☐ DEPLOY HAIR TIE TRICK
☐ BUY STRETCHY PANTS

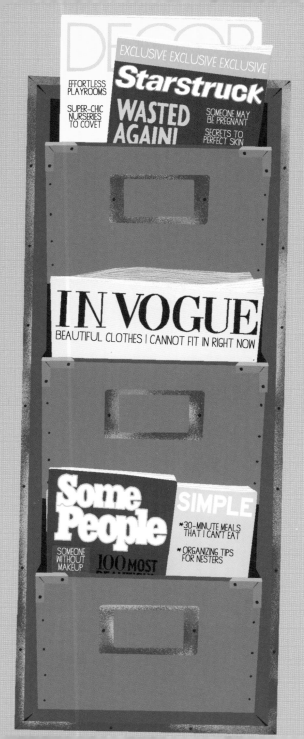

GUILTY PLEASURE:
GETTING TO APPOINTMENTS
EARLY TO INDULGE IN THE
LATEST STYLES & CELEBRITIES

- [ ]
- [ ]
- [ ]
- [ ]
- [ ]
- [ ]
- [ ]
- [ ]
- [ ]
- [ ]
- [ ]
- [ ]
- [ ]
- [ ]
- [ ]

IF THERE WAS EVER A TIME TO NAVEL-GAZE, IT'S NOW.

Week 3

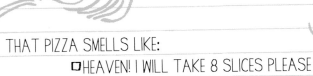

THAT PIZZA SMELLS LIKE:
☐ HEAVEN! I WILL TAKE 8 SLICES PLEASE
☐ DIRTY FEET AND I MUST GET OUT OF HERE

BABY IS THE SIZE
OF A PEPPERCORN

week 7

week 8

1
2
3
4
5
6
7
8

COMMENCE WEEK 8 OF FEELING DEBILITATED

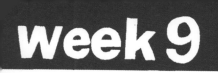
week 9

week 10

BABY IS THE SIZE
OF A KUMQUAT

week 11

THE VERY SWEETEST, MOST REASSURING SOUND

60 —	— 60
40 —	— 40
20 —	— 20
cm/s	cm
-20 —	— -2
-40 —	— -4
-60 —	— -6

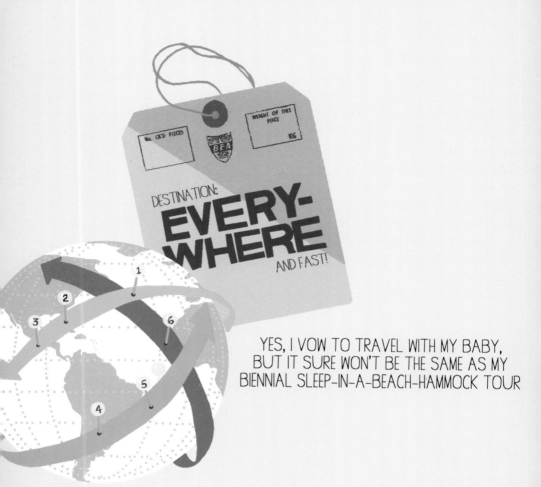

DESTINATION:

EVERY-WHERE

AND FAST!

YES, I VOW TO TRAVEL WITH MY BABY,
BUT IT SURE WON'T BE THE SAME AS MY
BIENNIAL SLEEP-IN-A-BEACH-HAMMOCK TOUR

2nd trimester

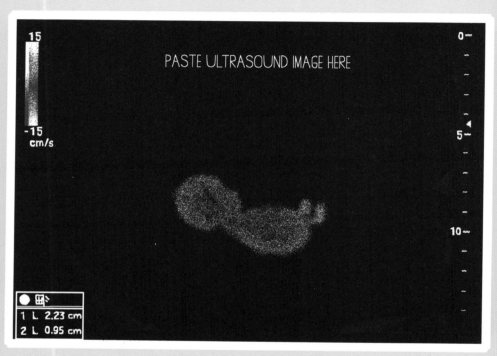

MY OH MY, HOW YOU'VE GROWN!

- [ ] ....
- [ ] ....
- [ ] ....
- [ ] ....
- [ ] ....
- [ ] ....
- [ ] ....
- [ ] ....
- [ ] ....
- [ ] ....
- [ ] ....
- [ ] ....
- [ ] ....
- [ ] ....
- [ ] ....

TELLING THE WORLD

FOLKS WE TOLD

HOW WE TOLD THEM

THEIR REACTIONS

BRING ON THE
CONFETTI

LET THE ADVICE ROLL IN!

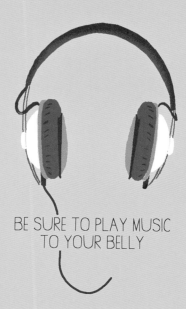

BE SURE TO PLAY MUSIC
TO YOUR BELLY

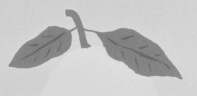

SMELL A LEMON WHEN
YOU FEEL QUEASY

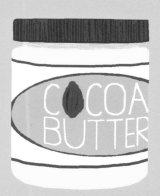

NIGHTLY SLATHERING OF
COCOA BUTTER WILL KEEP
STRETCH MARKS AT BAY

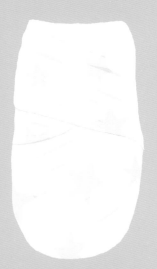

YOU ARE GOING TO NEED
THIS SPECIFIC SWADDLE

BEST ADVICE I'VE RECEIVED

- ☐ ....
- ☐ ....
- ☐ ....
- ☐ ....
- ☐ ....
- ☐ ....
- ☐ ....
- ☐ ....
- ☐ ....
- ☐ ....
- ☐ ....

FUNNIEST ADVICE I'VE HEARD

- ☐ ....
- ☐ ....
- ☐ ....
- ☐ ....
- ☐ ....
- ☐ ....
- ☐ ....
- ☐ ....
- ☐ ....
- ☐ ....
- ☐ ....

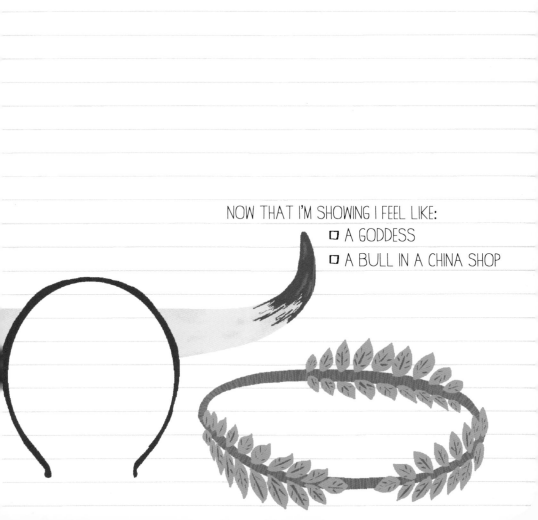

NOW THAT I'M SHOWING I FEEL LIKE:
- ☐ A GODDESS
- ☐ A BULL IN A CHINA SHOP

DEMI   FULL   EXTENDED

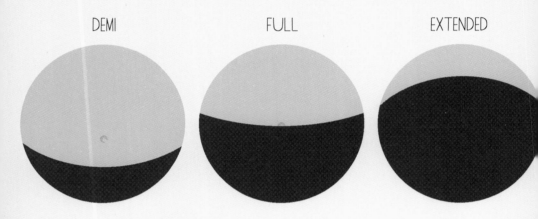

I DIDN'T KNOW IT WAS GOING TO BE THIS COMPLICATED

ALL THE CLOTHES I WILL NEED

- [ ]
- [ ]
- [ ]
- [ ]
- [ ]
- [ ]
- [ ]
- [ ]
- [ ]
- [ ]
- [ ]
- [ ]
- [ ]
- [ ]
- [ ]
- [ ]
- [ ]
- [ ]
- [ ]
- [ ]
- [ ]
- [ ]
- [ ]
- [ ]
- [ ]
- [ ]
- [ ]

DRAWINGS OF MY FOOD CRAVINGS

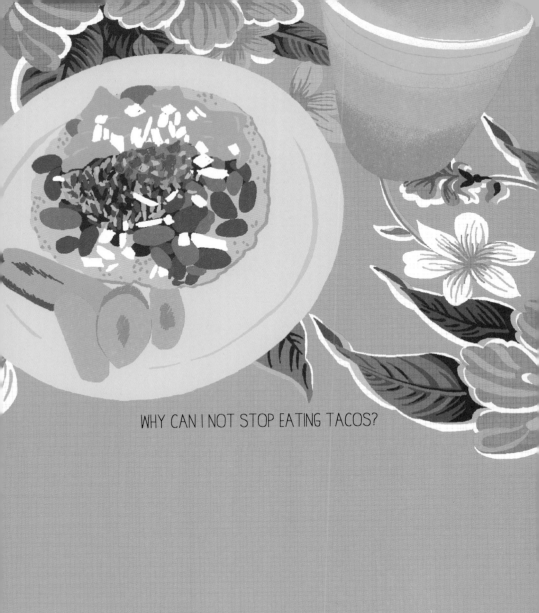

WHY CAN I NOT STOP EATING TACOS?

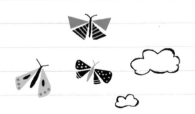

WERE THOSE FLUTTERS OR JUST GAS?

FOLKLORE METHODS OF PREDICTING THE SEX

IT'S A
girl

DULL PEE

BRIGHT PEE

IT'S A
boy

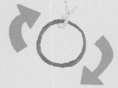

DANGLED RING
OVER BELLY SPINS

$$\begin{array}{r} 28 \\ +1 \\ \hline 29 \end{array}$$

AGE + MONTH
OF CONCEPTION
IS ODD #

$$\begin{array}{r} 35 \\ +3 \\ \hline 38 \end{array}$$

AGE + MONTH
OF CONCEPTION
IS EVEN #

DANGLED RING OVER
BELLY SWAYS
SIDE TO SIDE

MORNING SICKNESS

NO MORNING SICKNESS

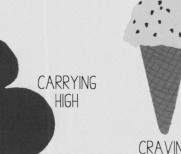

CARRYING
HIGH

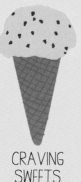

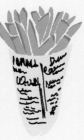

CARRYING
LOW

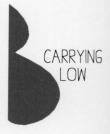

CRAVING
SWEETS

CRAVING
SALT

TO KNOW OR NOT TO KNOW
- ☐ TELL ME, TELL ME, TELL ME!
- ☐ SURPRISE ME LATER

I THINK I AM HAVING
- ☐ A LI'L DUDE
- ☐ A LI'L DUDETTE

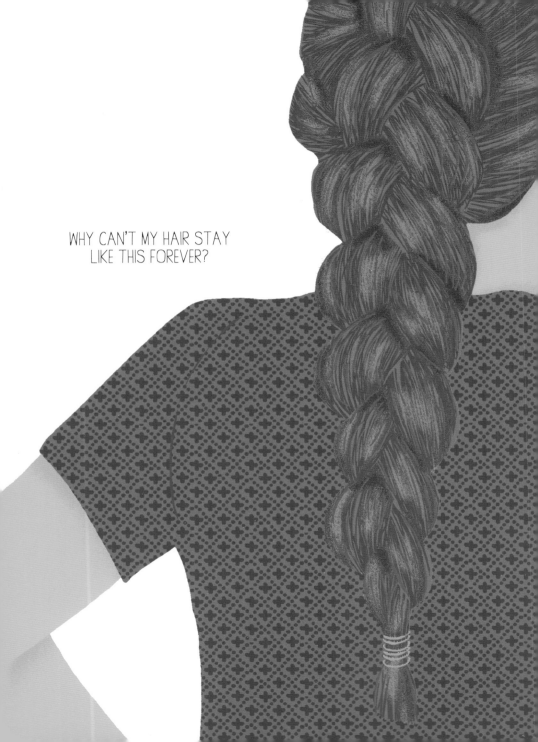

WHY CAN'T MY HAIR STAY
LIKE THIS FOREVER?

☐ THICK LIKE FARRAH FAWCETT'S
☐ SHINY LIKE BEYONCÉ'S

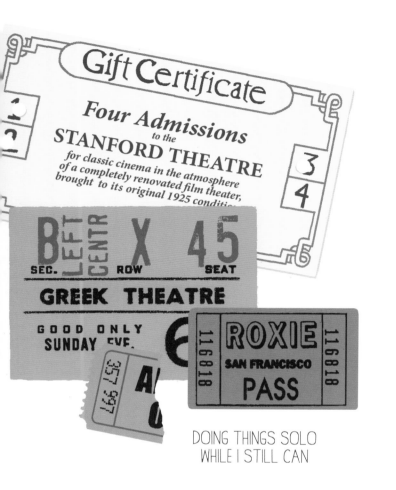

Gift Certificate

Four Admissions
to the
STANFORD THEATRE
for classic cinema in the atmosphere
of a completely renovated film theater,
brought to its original 1925 conditi...

3
4

SEC. B LEFT CENTR ROW X SEAT 45

GREEK THEATRE

GOOD ONLY
SUNDAY EVE.

ROXIE
SAN FRANCISCO
PASS

116818

116818

357 997

DOING THINGS SOLO
WHILE I STILL CAN

ADMIT
ONE

12813

- [ ]
- [ ]
- [ ]
- [ ]
- [ ]
- [ ]
- [ ]
- [ ]
- [ ]
- [ ]
- [ ]
- [ ]
- [ ]
- [ ]
- [ ]
- [ ]
- [ ]
- [ ]
- [ ]
- [ ]
- [ ]
- [ ]
- [ ]
- [ ]
- [ ]
- [ ]
- [ ]

FELLOW PASSENGERS GRACIOUSLY
OFFERING THEIR SEAT

1

⊘ DO NOT LEAN ON DOOR

⊘ DO NOT IGNORE PREGNANT WOMEN

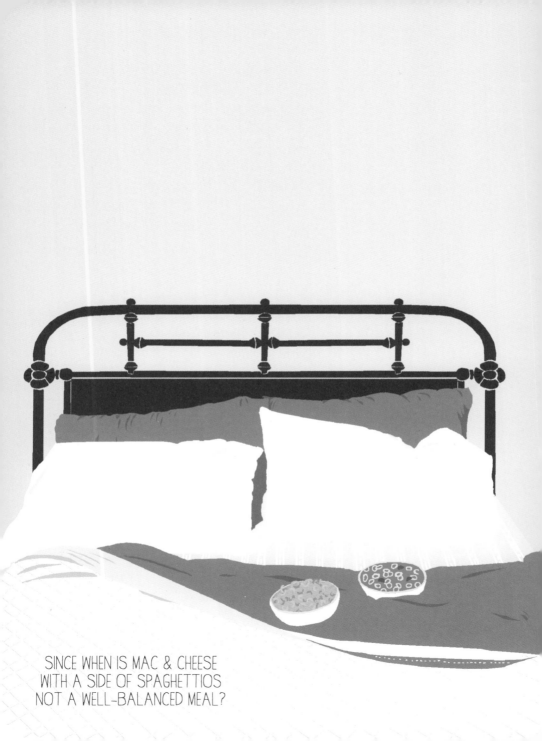

SINCE WHEN IS MAC & CHEESE
WITH A SIDE OF SPAGHETTIOS
NOT A WELL-BALANCED MEAL?

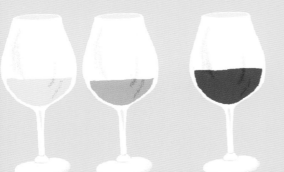

MISSING THE LITTLE THINGS
☐ HAPPY HOUR
☐ NORMAL-SIZED BLADDER
☐ CUTE SHOES
☐ FRILLY BRAS
☐ _____

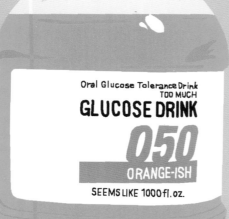

Oral Glucose Tolerance Drink
TOO MUCH
GLUCOSE DRINK
050
ORANGE-ISH
SEEMS LIKE 1000 fl. oz.

GIVING BIRTH IS BOUND TO
BE MORE ENJOYABLE THAN
THE GLUCOSE TEST

- [ ]
- [ ]
- [ ]
- [ ]
- [ ]
- [ ]
- [ ]
- [ ]
- [ ]
- [ ]
- [ ]
- [ ]
- [ ]
- [ ]
- [ ]

week 13

ALL THIS NAVEL-GAZING IS MAKING ME HUNGRY.

week 15

week 16

THE DAY I FOUND STRETCHY PANTS I THOUGHT:
- ☐ WHERE HAVE YOU BEEN ALL MY LIFE?
- ☐ LIFE AS I KNOW IT IS CLEARLY OVER

week 17

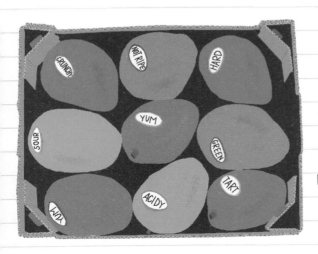

INEXPLICABLE CRAVINGS
CONTINUE...DEVOURING
UNRIPE CRUNCHY MANGOES
BY THE FLAT

week 19

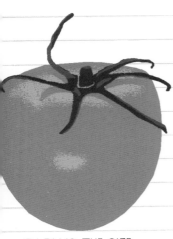

BABY IS THE SIZE
OF A TOMATO

week 21

COMBATING THE DREADED LEG CRAMP

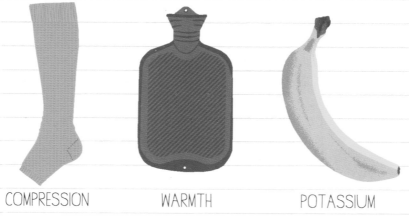

COMPRESSION   WARMTH   POTASSIUM

week 24

I EXPECT MY LIFE IS GOING TO CHANGE:
- ☐ IN EVERY WAY POSSIBLE
- ☐ NOT AS MUCH AS EVERYONE SAYS

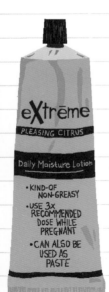

eXtrēme
PLEASING CITRUS

Daily Moisture Lotion

• KIND-OF
  NON-GREASY
• USE 3x
  RECOMMENDED
  DOSE WHILE
  PREGNANT
• CAN ALSO BE
  USED AS
  PASTE

CANNOT GET ENOUGH MOISTURE!

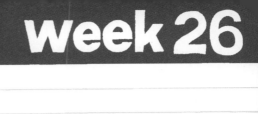
week 26

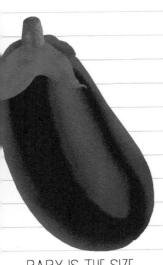

BABY IS THE SIZE
OF AN EGGPLANT

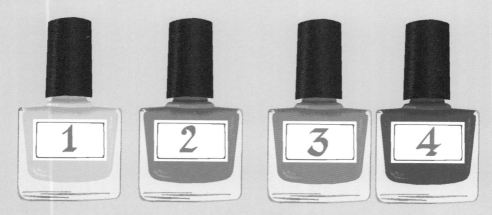

NOW THAT I CAN'T REACH MY TOES, I REALLY
WISH THE MANI-PEDI PLACE HAD A PUNCH CARD

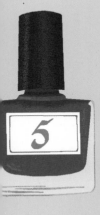

3rd
trimester

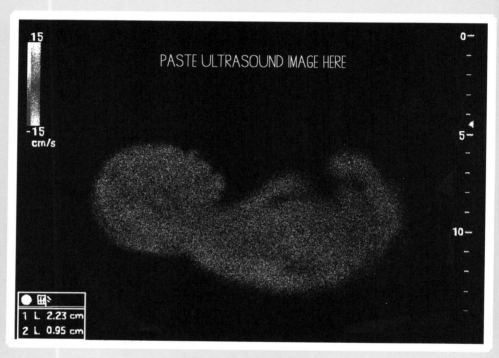

CAN'T WAIT TO MEET YOU!

- [ ]
- [ ]
- [ ]
- [ ]
- [ ]
- [ ]
- [ ]
- [ ]
- [ ]
- [ ]
- [ ]
- [ ]
- [ ]
- [ ]
- [ ]

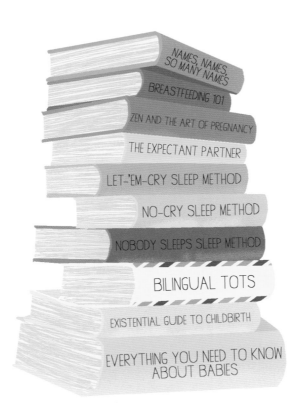

NAMES, NAMES, SO MANY NAMES

BREASTFEEDING 101

ZEN AND THE ART OF PREGNANCY

THE EXPECTANT PARTNER

LET-'EM-CRY SLEEP METHOD

NO-CRY SLEEP METHOD

NOBODY SLEEPS SLEEP METHOD

BILINGUAL TOTS

EXISTENTIAL GUIDE TO CHILDBIRTH

EVERYTHING YOU NEED TO KNOW ABOUT BABIES

GOING BACK TO SCHOOL

BOOKS TO READ

- [ ]
- [ ]
- [ ]
- [ ]
- [ ]
- [ ]
- [ ]
- [ ]
- [ ]
- [ ]
- [ ]

CLASSES TO SIGN UP FOR

- [ ]
- [ ]
- [ ]
- [ ]
- [ ]
- [ ]
- [ ]
- [ ]
- [ ]
- [ ]
- [ ]

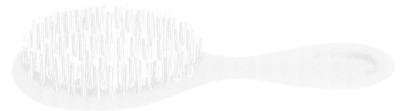

PREPARE

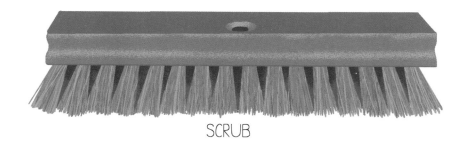

SCRUB

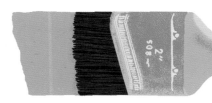

PRETTIFY

THE NEED TO NEST

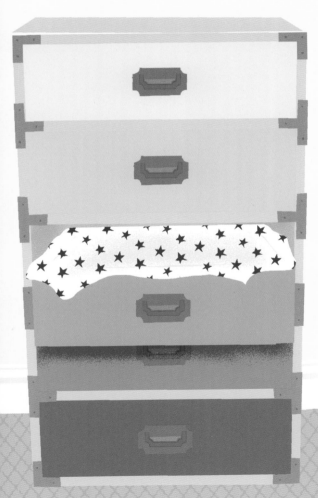

MY GRANDMA SAYS ALL
I NEED IS A BLANKET
AND A DRESSER DRAWER

NICKNAME

CRITTER - MOST OF THE TIME
CREATURE - ON OCCASION
NUGGET - SOMETIMES
PEA - ONCE IN AWHILE

ADELINE - MATERNAL GRANDMA
SOFIA - PATERNAL GRANDMA
ROSE - GREAT-AUNT
SLOAN - SOLID NAME

FRANK - PATERNAL GRANDPA
          & MATERNAL UNCLE
OLE - JUST LIKE THE SOUND OF IT
AI - HAWAIIAN MEANING SEA

THINGS WE ARE THINKING OF CALLING YOU LATER

FIRST NAME   SPECIAL MEANING

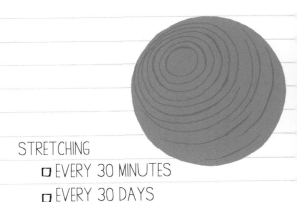

STRETCHING
- ☐ EVERY 30 MINUTES
- ☐ EVERY 30 DAYS

WALKING
- ☐ TO THE FRIDGE
- ☐ TO CURE RESTLESSNESS

SWIMMING
- ☐ MAGICAL WEIGHTLESSNESS
- ☐ SWIMSUIT? NOT A CHANCE!

KEGEL EXERCISES
- ☐ DOING THEM
- ☐ KNOW I SHOULD BE DOING THEM

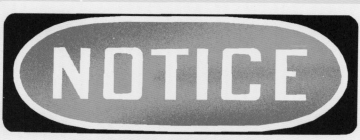

NOTICE

STRONG MAGNETIC
BELLY ALWAYS ON
UNAUTHORIZED PERSONNEL
– *KEEP OFF* –

SOMEONE JUST TOUCHED MY BELLY WITHOUT ASKING

- [ ] ....
- [ ] ....
- [ ] ....
- [ ] ....
- [ ] ....
- [ ] ....
- [ ] ....
- [ ] ....
- [ ] ....
- [ ] ....
- [ ] ....
- [ ] ....
- [ ] ....
- [ ] ....
- [ ] ....
- [ ] ....
- [ ] ....
- [ ] ....
- [ ] ....
- [ ] ....
- [ ] ....
- [ ] ....
- [ ] ....
- [ ] ....
- [ ] ....
- [ ] ....

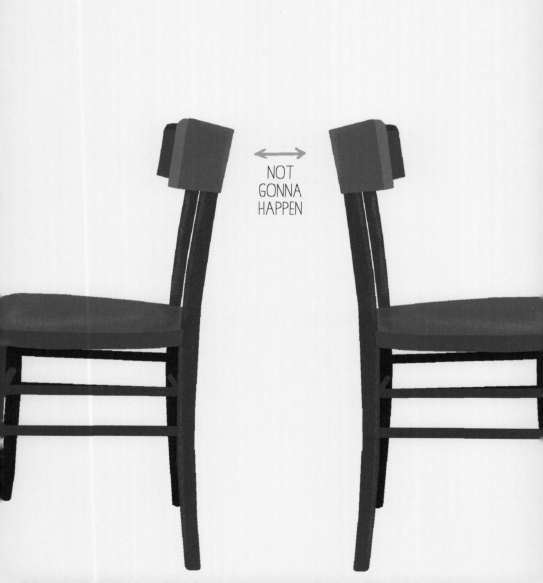

TODAY I COULD NO LONGER FIT:
- ☐ BETWEEN THE CAFÉ CHAIRS
- ☐ BEHIND THE STEERING WHEEL
- ☐ THROUGH THE SUBWAY TURNSTILE
- ☐ _____

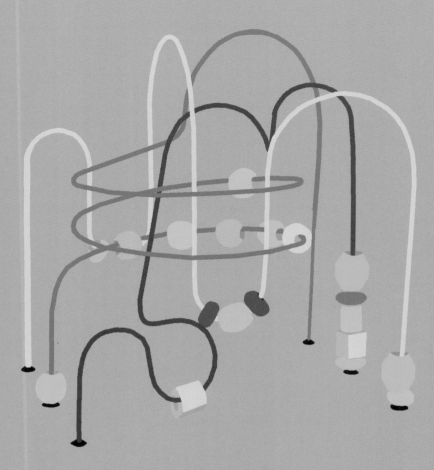

QUIETLY FREAKING OUT ABOUT PARENTING WHILE
WATCHING A 3-YEAR-OLD FOR THE AFTERNOON

I AM FEELING:

___% OVERWHELMED

___% ECSTATIC

GO-TO MATERNITY OUTFIT:

_____

OUTFIT I CANNOT WAIT TO BURN:

_____

__ # OF CONSECUTIVE DAYS WEARING THE SAME PANTS

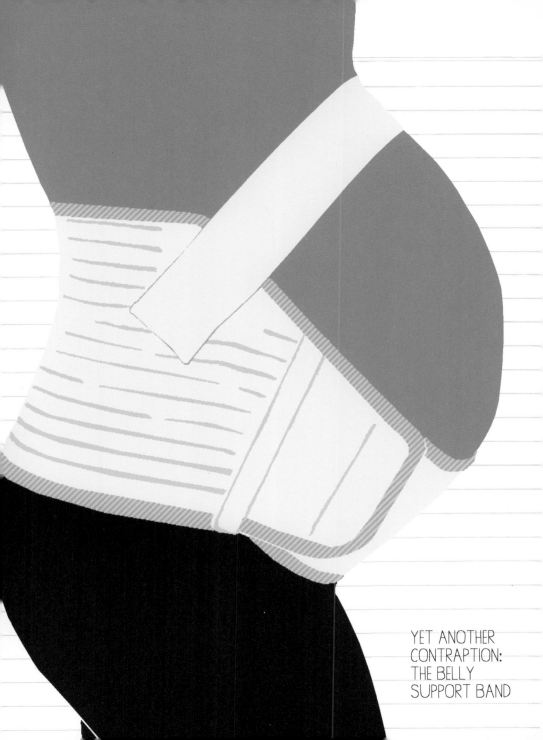

YET ANOTHER
CONTRAPTION:
THE BELLY
SUPPORT BAND

KICK COUNTS	SUN	MON	TUES
WEEK # ___ TIME			
MINUTES TO REACH 10			
# ___ TIME			
MINUTES TO REACH 10			
# ___ TIME			
MINUTES TO REACH 10			
# ___ TIME			
MINUTES TO REACH 10			
# ___ TIME			
MINUTES TO REACH 10			
# ___ TIME			
MINUTES TO REACH 10			
# ___ TIME			
MINUTES TO REACH 10			
# ___ TIME			
MINUTES TO REACH 10			
# ___ TIME			
MINUTES TO REACH 10			
# ___ TIME			
MINUTES TO REACH 10			
# ___ TIME			
MINUTES TO REACH 10			
# ___ TIME			
MINUTES TO REACH 10			
# ___ TIME			
MINUTES TO REACH 10			

WED	THURS	FRI	SAT

I'M PRETTY SURE THAT WAS JUST AN ELBOW

SLEEP IS BUT A FAINT MEMORY

THE WEDGE

THE STANDARD

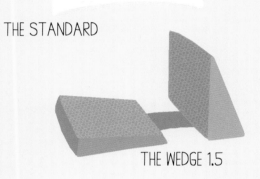

THE WEDGE 1.5

THE SNOOGLE

THE WEDGE 2.0

THE CONTOUR

THE BODY

- [ ]
- [ ]
- [ ]
- [ ]
- [ ]
- [ ]
- [ ]
- [ ]
- [ ]
- [ ]
- [ ]
- [ ]
- [ ]
- [ ]
- [ ]
- [ ]
- [ ]
- [ ]
- [ ]
- [ ]
- [ ]
- [ ]
- [ ]
- [ ]
- [ ]
- [ ]
- [ ]

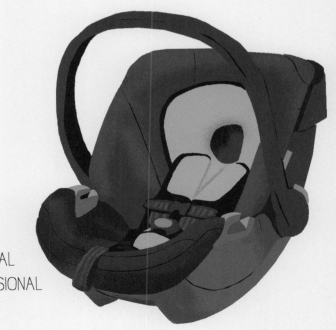

GOING TO NEED TO:

    ☐ STUDY THE MANUAL

    ☐ CALL IN A PROFESSIONAL

FOLKLORE TIDBIT#372

IF YOU HAVE HEARTBURN THAT MEANS
THE BABY HAS A LOT OF HAIR

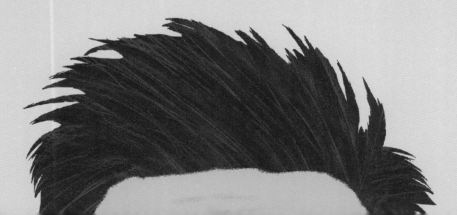

week 29

MY NAVEL IS GETTING HARDER TO FIND FOR GAZING.

week 30

MY BELLY LOOKS LIKE A:
- ☐ PEAR
- ☐ BASKETBALL

week 31

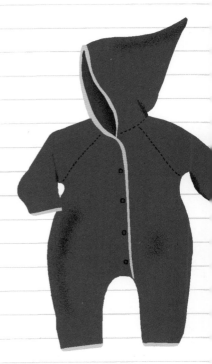

OUTFITS THAT TURN THE
BABY INTO A TINY ELF?
I AM CERTAIN TO SPEND
MY SAVINGS ON BABY
CLOTHES

week 33

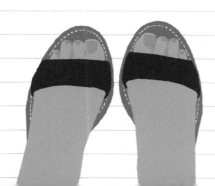

SO SWOLLEN
MY ANKLES
WENT MISSING

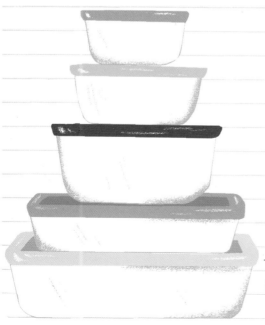

STOCKPILING
FROZEN MEALS
TO EAT ONCE TIME IS
NO LONGER MY OWN

week 37

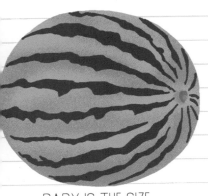

BABY IS THE SIZE
OF A WATERMELON

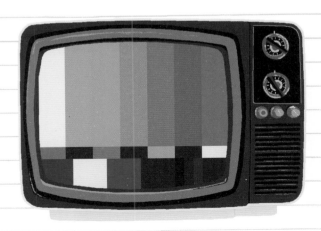

EVEN WATCHING TV TAKES TOO MUCH ENERGY

THE DAY I WENT INTO LABOR

WHERE I WAS WHEN
MY WATER BROKE:

KEPT MY COOL
OR FREAKED OUT:

ITEMS THAT HELPED EASE
THE CONTRACTIONS: . . . .

. . . .

ALL AS EXPECTED
OR CHANGE IN PLANS: . . . .

. . . .

PURE BLISS SHORT-LIVED & WELL WORTH IT EASIER THAN EXPECTED YIKES, THAT HURT

LABOR PAIN-O-METER

NOTES FROM THE BIRTH

WHERE YOU WERE BORN: ....

DOCTOR OR MIDWIFE: ....

NURSE OR DOULA: ....

WHO CUT THE CORD: ....

WHO WAS BESIDE ME: ....

☐ ....
☐ ....
☐ ....
☐ ....
☐ ....
☐ ....
☐ ....
☐ ....
☐ ....
☐ ....
☐ ....
☐ ....
☐ ....
☐ ....
☐ ....
☐ ....
☐ ....
☐ ....
☐ ....
☐ ....
☐ ....
☐ ....
☐ ....
☐ ....

HOW WILL I
FIND THE TIME
FOR PROPER
THANK-YOUS?

THANK
THANK
THANK